Ageless Remedies from Mother's Kitchen

Rediscovered and Collected
by
Hanna Kroeger

4th Edition

About the Author

Hanna Kroeger is a daughter of a German missionary. She studied nursing at the University of Freiburg, Germany, and worked in a hospital for natural healing under Professor Brauchle.

In 1953 she and her family came to America. In 1958 she started a health food store.

Hanna has authored many books. In her summer retreat, "Peaceful Meadow," and her church connected to it, the "Chapel of Miracles," she is teaching and sharing.

I dedicate this book to the mothers of this nation.
They are the torchbearers to a healthier future.
–Hanna Kroeger

Introduction

The knowledge of the amazing therapeutic values in foods becomes the focal point of this booklet.

With the hundreds and hundreds of drugs on the market, mothers still go to the kitchen and prepare specific foods for the sick. Mothers apply liniments and compresses, mothers concoct teas out of spices and herbs. Why do they go to all the trouble when a "pill" as recommended should do?

These old recipes work without danger of poisoning the system. These recipes are effective, they are handed down from mothers to daughters. These recipes are at hand and, with the economic loss in every pocket, they are inexpensive. Mothers have a sixth sense for healing and are naturally able to take away the misery of a sickness. This booklet is your guideline, the tools are in your kitchen.

I ask you readers, whenever you have a special recipe from your kitchen that helps in a specific way, share with all of us.

With this method of sharing we will have a healthier nation soon.

A

ABDOMEN
Distended without nausea
> Nutmeg.

ABDOMINAL TENDERNESS
Linden flower tea

H-12
> Place on navel.

ABSENCE OF ALL MORAL RESTRAINT
Anacardium occidentale (cashew nut)

ACHING OF HEELS
Hot pepper
> If hot peppers upset your stomach, sprinkle hot peppers on the soles of your feet and put on your socks. Hot peppers and radishes contain benzene which is needed for proper functioning of feet and sinuses.

ACID DYSPEPSIA
Raw potatoes
> Eat a piece of raw potato before each meal.

ACNE
Buttermilk and honey
> Boil buttermilk and, when thickened, add honey so it becomes a thick cream. Apply wherever needed.

(*See also* PIMPLES)

ADRENAL GLAND FOOD
Alfalfa seed
> 1 tablespoon seeds.

PABA
> 2 tablets PABA.

Licorice root
> Make tea or chew the root.

Protein
> More protein needed.

Dates and sunflower seed drink

AGING
Keeps old age away
> Thyme
> Lavender
> *H-12*

Whey
> Premature aging is a mineral deficiency. Whey is such a good helper in your kitchen. It has a lot of minerals. It is a remedy that will keep your muscles young. It will keep your joints moveable and ligaments elastic. When age wants to bend your back take whey.

AIR/CAR/SEASICKNESS
> Cover solar plexus with newspaper. In less than 10 minutes, relief.

ALCOHOL
Cucumber
> Give cucumber to someone who drank too much alcohol. It will reduce the alcohol's intoxicating effect. Cucumber has an enzyme called erepsin.

Vitamin B_1
> 100 mg 3 times daily.

Honey
> Something in honey removes alcohol from the blood extra fast.

ALCOHOLISM
> is candida encased in liver.

ALLERGEN
Watercress

> Watercress is extremely valuable since it is full of vitamins E, B, and C. It is an antiallergen and should be more widely used. Watercress is often used to decorate salads, sandwiches, and sauces. When eaten by itself, give only small portions since it is potent.

ALLERGIC TO WOOL
Magnesium

ALLERGY
Orange rind

> Orange rind or peelings are such good allergy relievers. The stuffed up nose and clogged up air passages open up and healthful sleep can be expected.

Sage

> Tastes best on a piece of buttered whole grain bread (rye or wheat). Sage—*salvia officinalis*—the Latin word *salvia* means healing, being healthy.

Banana

> For energy and nerves, hinders allergies.

A, B_{12}, E, G, pantothenic acid, L-histidine

ALONE, DESIRE TO BE
Cayenne pepper

ANEMIC

> Always remove worms first. Beet juice and yellow dock have iron.

Grape juice, blackstrap molasses

> 2 teaspoons blackstrap molasses in 1 glass grape juice.

Grape juice

> 1 glass grape juice and 1 egg yolk.

Wine

> $\frac{1}{2}$ glass red wine, $\frac{1}{2}$ glass water, 2 egg yolks

Spinach

> Blood builder, raw is best.

Raisins and grapefruit
> 2 ounces dark raisins 3 times daily for 1 day. ½ grapefruit 2 times daily second day. Alternate raisins and grapefruit for 3 weeks to make you strong and resistant to disease.

(*See also* SPLEEN)

ANGINA PECTORIS
Apple cider vinegar
> When angina hits suddenly, rush to the kitchen to heat apple cider vinegar. Take a Turkish towel and wet it with the warm vinegar. Apply to the back and chest of angina sufferer until help arrives.

ANTIBIOTIC
Avocado seeds
> Seeds of an avocado contain antibiotic. Pound seed and make a tea.

ANTISEPTIC
Lemon
> Lemon juice is nature's most powerful antiseptic. Use it externally on sores, corns, and dandruff, and gargle with it. Drink plenty of lemon juice when fever hits.

ANTISPASMODIC
Caraway
> This is a very well-known spice. It is antispasmodic, improves appetite, subsides gastric distention, takes out phlegm, and is useful for stomach disorders. It mainly works on the stomach.

ANTI-TOBACCO
Apple
> Detoxifying as anti-tobacco.

ANTI-TUMOR
Garlic
> A natural antibiotic, anti-tumor garlic has M-rays to search out harmful agents.

ANUS
Painful
> Ginger tea.

APPETITE IN CHILDREN
Lack of
> Cranberries as juice or as a sauce.

ARTERIES
Yogurt and applesauce
> 1 dish a day to keep arteries clean.

ARTERIES, HARDENING
> Brussels sprouts, alfalfa, garlic, vitamin F, whey, violet, hyssop, clover. 4 cups per day.

Parsley
> A good food to keep arteries clear.

Indian remedy
> Tea of sassafras. Also ½ teaspoon cream of tartar 2 times per week.

ARTHRITIS
Brown paper
> Take brown paper and make layers of it. Sew this paper between two layers of flannel and use it as a bed covering. The DMSO pine residue will relieve the pain and heal.

Celery, parsley, and celeriac
> When you come down with arthritis, eat celery and parsley every day or juice them and eat celeriac.

Whey
> Mix 2 tablespoons whey with 1 tablespoon lecithin, mix in 8 tablespoons of vegetable broth. Do this 3 times daily for several months.

Avocado seed
> Pound avocado seed, make a strong tea, and apply to skin.

Swiss chard
> (Contains Wulzen factor.)

Garlic
> Crush garlic, spread in cloth like butter on bread. Wrap poultice around arthritic joint 2 to 12 hours, which will raise a large burn blister full of water. This will break and run out, drawing the disease out of the joint. Now heal up the burn with aloe vera juice and see amazing results.

Apple cider vinegar, honey, water

> 2 teaspoons vinegar, 2 teaspoons honey, and 8 ounces water together are a good cleansing remedy for arthritis. Take it 3 times daily with meals.

Check alkalinity

> When too much acid, add phosphorus and magnesium to your diet. When too alkaline, add calcium and protein.

Lemon, orange, grapefruit

> Grate up 1 lemon, 1 orange, and 1 grapefruit. Add 2 teaspoons of cream of tartar, add 2 tablespoons Epsom salts, add 1 quart water. Drink 2 ounces 3 times per day.

Five foods

> Black cherries as juice.
> Alfalfa seeds or juice or tablets.
> Peanut oil, 2 tablespoons.
> Celeriac or celery root as a dish.
> Liquid rice B-complex.

ASTHMA

Sunflower seeds

> Take 1 quart of sunflower seeds, put in $1/2$ gallon water, boil down to 1 quart of water, strain, add 1 pint of honey, and boil down to a syrup. 1 teaspoon 3 times daily is the dose.

Radish and honey

> Grate black radish and add honey to it. Before going to bed take 1 teaspoon of the mixture. Go on a $1/2$ day fast. The time you do not eat, take 2 quarts of water, soak green pineapples in it, and let sit for 2 hours. Drink from that fluid for the other half of the day all you want. Do this for 10 to 14 days.

Lemon juice

> 2 tablespoons lemon juice before each meal.

Thyme

> Thyme powdered and mixed with honey. 1 teaspoon every hour.
>
> OR
>
> Red onion, raw, juice mixed with raw sugar. 1 teaspoon every hour.
>
> Wild plum bark, wild cherry bark.

Asthma without anxiety
    Ginger.

Asthma attack
    Put hands in hot water.

Cranberry juice
    Concentrated cranberry for asthma. You may get it at your favorite health food store or prepare it yourself: 1 pound cranberries, 1 pint water. Boil until cranberries are done, then keep it in refrigerator. Dosage: 1 teaspoon.

ASTIGMATISM (myopic)
Tiger lily

ATHLETE'S FOOT
Vitamin A
    Bathe feet in rosehips tea or lemon juice or follow suggestions on your Clorox bottle.

Spinach seed and onion seed
    Simmer 2 tablespoons of the seeds in 1 quart water for $\frac{1}{2}$ hour, then soak feet in the water.

B

B$_{17}$ (homemade)
Apricot, apricot kernels
> 4 apricot kernels, 2 pieces dried apricot, limewater or *Calcarea Carbonica*. 2 times daily.

BABIES
Milk
> Mama's milk best, goat's milk next best. Ripe banana and ripe coconut ground and squeezed very good.

BACKACHE
Affecting hips and sacrum, has to walk stooping
> Chestnut.

Children
> Alfalfa seed, dill seed.

BACKWARD CHILDREN
Alfalfa seed
> Sprouted.

Dill
> Seasoning.

Bran
> Pour 8 ounces of boiling water over 1 tablespoon bran. Add honey to taste and give this to children, invalids, and mentally disturbed people.

BEE STING

In the mouth or throat: this is a serious accident

Take 1 teaspoon of salt and put it in the mouth at once. It has helped many from strangling to death.

Onion

Rub on raw onion.

BILE

Increase bile

Black garden radish

Bile duct sluggish

Mugwort: $\frac{1}{2}$ cup tea, a strong herb.

Artichoke

Brings a clear urine and increases the flow of bile. Tones up the liver. Claims are made that it keeps the arteries smooth and a person free from weak digestion. It is useful for albumin in the urine and for jaundice.

Soup

A small bowl of soup at the beginning of the meal is stimulating to the bile.

BIRTHMARKS

Apply castor oil

Takes several months to make them disappear.

BLACKHEADS

Cucumber

Cut a piece of cucumber and rub it over your face. You can also cover your face with cucumber peelings, the cut side to the skin.

Strawberries

Rub fresh strawberries over your face.

Wash

Wash face with hot water and then sprinkle with cold water.

Vitamin A is needed

Soap

Use soap and water, lathering freely; dry, rinse thoroughly. Afterwards sponge with witch hazel daily.

BLADDER PAIN
Marshmallow root
> Due to a cold: 1 tablespoon marshmallow root in 1 cup water. Drink hot.

Pomegranate
> As a juice $\frac{1}{2}$ cup with $\frac{1}{2}$ cup water, or better as a fruit eat 1 twice a day.

BLADDER STONES
Carrot leaves, parsley tea
> 1 quart a day for 3 days, then just 2 cups a day.

BLADDER TROUBLE
Steamed parsley

Pomegranate
> As a juice $\frac{1}{2}$ cup with $\frac{1}{2}$ cup water, or better as a fruit eat 1 twice a day.

Pumpkin seed
> Pumpkin seed is specific for strengthening the bladder muscle. Take 1 teaspoon 3 times daily or more if desired.

BLADDER, WEAK
Pumpkin seed
> Pumpkin seed is specific for strengthening the bladder muscle. Take 1 teaspoon 3 times daily or more if desired.

Chickpea

BLEEDING, BOWELS
Cinnamon tea
> $\frac{1}{2}$ cup, 4 times daily.

BLEEDING CUTS
> Cover the cut with unglazed brown paper wetted with vinegar.

BLEEDING (female)
Okra

(*See* FEMALE BLEEDING)

BLEEDING GUMS

Old-time recipe for bleeding gums and breaking capillaries: Wash and cut 6 lemons in little pieces. Cover with 1½ quarts water and bring to boil. Turn off the heat and let sit for 25 minutes. Strain and set aside until cool. Take 6 ounces 2 times daily for 10 days. In case of bleeding gums, hold juice in your mouth also.

Papaya seeds

Chew 1 teaspoon papaya seeds 4 times daily and spit out after chewing thoroughly.

Black pepper

Black pepper freshly ground is loaded with chromium which is needed for proper functioning of the pancreas and heart.

(*See also* GUMS)

BLEEDING TOOTH

After extraction

Moisten 1 tea bag (black tea) with warm water and apply.

BLOATEDNESS

Sage tea

Fennel

BLOATING

Caraway and fennel

Take equal parts, grind seeds in your blender.

Sage

Sage with peppermint as a tea.

In children and adults

1 teaspoon fennel. Bring to a boil in 8 ounces water. Simmer 10 minutes. Strain 1 to 2 cups for adult, children ½ cup.

BLOOD BUILDERS

Egg yolk

Egg yolk mixed in some concord grape juice is a terrific blood builder.

Apricots

Eat 2 dried apricots 2 times daily or soak them and blend them.

Blackstrap molasses

2 to 4 teaspoons daily.

Beet and grape juice
> 1 part red beet juice, 2 parts dark grape juice. Take 2 tablespoons 3 times daily.

BLOOD CLEANSER
Lemon juice, honey, and water
> 6 ounces every 2 hours.

BLOOD POISONING
Cranberries
> Boil 1 quart cranberry juice with 8 cloves and 1 teaspoon cinnamon. Add 1 quart of water and drink this in a day.

BLOOD PRESSURE
Parsley
> Make a parsley tea and also add parsley to salads and soups.

Turnip tops
> Boil turnip tops as you would eat spinach, eat with rice. Once every day will lower the blood pressure.

Parsley, celery, garlic
> Eat plenty of parsley and add garlic and celery. Better yet, buy a juicer, juice the vegetables, and drink 6 ounces 2 times daily.

Lecithin, B_{12}, B-complex, garlic
> For the elasticity of the vessels.

Apples
> 2 apples a day will do it. Dr. Ancel Keys' research proved it.

Watermelon seeds
> Watermelon seeds dilate the blood vessels, lower blood pressure, and improve kidney function.

BLOOD PRESSURE—HIGH
Oranges and lemons
> 3 oranges, 2 lemons. Cut into pieces. Boil in 1 quart of water for 15 minutes. Then add 2 tablespoons of honey. Boil another 10 minutes. Strain and drink 6 ounces 3 times daily before meals (not for diabetics). Oftentimes the kidney diet does miracles for the high blood pressure sufferer.

Lecithin, B_1, B-complex, garlic
> For the elasticity of the vessels.

BLOOD PRESSURE—LOW
Pepper
> Add cayenne pepper to your food.

Apricots
> Mix apricots and dark raisins. Eat 2 tablespoons 3 times daily.

Protein

BLOOD PURIFIER
Beets, carrots, cranberries, cucumber

Strawberry leaves
> For skin.

BLOOD THINNERS
Rosemary and red clover
> Red clover tea—leaves.
> Red clover tea—seeds (stronger).

BLOOD TOXINS
Cranberries
> Boil 1 quart cranberry juice with 8 cloves and 1 teaspoon cinnamon. Add 1 quart of water and drink this in a day.

BODY ODOR
Chlorophyll
> Everything that is green has chlorophyll. Take plenty of green drinks or buy liquid chlorophyll to combat body odor.

BOILS
Onion
> Put onion poultice over a boil to bring it to a head.

Indian remedy
> To bring boil to head, cut stem out of ripe tomato, turn tomato over boil.

BOILS AND PIMPLES
Nutmeg
> Combine $^1/_3$ teaspoon nutmeg (freshly ground), 1 teaspoon honey, and 4 to 5 ounces hot water. Drink this for 3 mornings in a row. Don't drink it for 3 days. Repeat this 9 times.

(*See also* PIMPLES)

BOOSTER

Chia seed, sunflower seed, sesame seed, flax seed

> Mix equal portions of each and soak 1 tablespoon overnight in $^1\!/_2$ glass of water. Next morning add $^1\!/_2$ glass juice or more. Drink this once a day and you will have plenty of energy.

(*See also* PEP DRINK)

BOTULISM

> 2 teaspoons vinegar in 7 ounces water every hour 4 to 6 times.

BOWELS, CLEANSING OF

When lots of gas

> 1 quart hot water with 1 tablespoon of molasses and juice of 1 lemon.

Flax seed

> Flax seed must be gently simmered for, say, $^1\!/_2$ hour and allowed to stand where it will remain hot for 1 or 2 hours longer. Put 2 tablespoons in 2 cups of boiling water; let it boil down to 1 cup. Add a little sugar to taste. The juice of $^1\!/_2$ lemon makes a tasty addition. Drink the whole cupful at bedtime and swallow all the seeds. The mucilage is soothing to the bowels and, in combination with the seeds, often produces a good bowel movement. Excellent to take about once a week, every 4 days, or more often if needed. It is harmless.

BOWELS, DROPPED

Prickly pear

BRAIN FOOD

> 1 pound sunflower seeds, $^1\!/_4$ pound almonds, 1 pound wheat. Grind up and eat 2 heaping tablespoons a day.

Barley and coconut

> Brain cocktail: 1 cup barley, 1 cup coconut juice, 1 tablespoon lecithin. Honey if desired.

Coconut

> Coconut meat is a brain food. Eat the meat and drink the milk.

Cardamom

> Cardamom is an eye and brain food.

Leek

> Cut leeks, boil, and use in soups or in salads.

BRAIN TUMOR

Shave head, apply tofu over head, and change the compress when tofu gets yellow. Or raw crushed tomato in cheesecloth poultice.

BREAST CAKED AND SORE

Carrots

Grate raw carrots and apply to hardened and sore breast.

Lumps or pain

Bag balm available at veterinary supply house.

Breast, knots in

Grate carrots and make a poultice over breast.
Simmer laurel leaves in oil and apply to breast gently without pressure.

Sticky pain in left breast

Myrtle as a tea.

BREATH, SHORTNESS OF

Red onion juice

Bring to a boil, add honey, simmer for 15 minutes. Take 1 teaspoon every hour.

1 tablespoon raw onion juice on 1 teaspoon sugar.

Black tea

A cup of black tea often removes breathing difficulty until you find doctor's help.

BRIGHT'S DISEASE (kidney trouble)

Watermelon seed tea

Watermelon and its seeds. For 2 days, eat nothing but watermelon. Eat watermelon always by itself.

(*See also* KIDNEY INFLAMMATION)

BROMIDE POISON (or narcotic poisoning)

Coffee

Give strong coffee by mouth or as an enema when someone has taken an overdose of bromide. 1 cup every hour. When in stupor make coffee enema every half hour.

BRONCHITIS
Flax seed

> To 1 pint of flax seed tea, add the juice of 2 lemons, add 3 tablespoons honey. Take 1 teaspoon every half hour until relieved.

BRUISES
Tobacco

> Moisten tobacco and slap over bruise. It will burn but, when the burn leaves, you can continue to work.

BURNS
Cold water

> Place under cold water until all pain is gone

> Some dip a burn in cold fresh cream, if available.

Black tea

Egg white

> Egg white slightly beaten and applied to first- and second-degree burns will take away the pain.

C and E

Burning feet

> B_6, B-complex, pantothenic acid, E, copper, iron.

Burning pains

> B_{12}.

Burning sensation in body and limbs

> Manganese
> B_{12}.

Burning of skin with itching

> Homeopathic *Ranunculus bulbosus* (buttercup).

Burning of alimentary canal

> *Iris versicolor* (blue flag).

Burning pains

> Cayenne pepper, *H-12*.

C

CALCIUM SUPPLIER
Broccoli
> Broccoli has more available calcium than milk or other sources. Broccoli supplies calcium to the system.

Cauliflower
> A very good calcium supplier.

CANKER SORES
Canker sores in mouth
> Use sage tea for mouth sores (or sore eyes). Or apply 1 inch of powdered sage against the sore. Or apply goldenseal powder or raw onion.

CAPILLARY FRAGILITY
> Cut 3 lemons into small pieces, add the peelings of 3 more lemons cut small. Boil in $1^1/_2$ quarts of water for 20 minutes. Steep for 25 minutes, strain drink. 1 cup 2 times daily for 2 weeks.

CATARACTS
> Equal parts yellow onion juice with honey. Mix well. 1 or 2 drops into eye 2 times a day.

Coconut
> Take the fresh juice from a coconut and with an eye dropper apply as much as the eye can hold, then apply hot wet cloths over the eye. Keep patient lying down and keep the towels hot for 10 minutes.

Natural Cheddar cheese, sage honey

Eat 2 ounces of Cheddar cheese 2 times daily, drop 1 drop of sage honey in each eye.

A doctor in the East gives vitamin B_2 against cataracts with excellent results.

Bean pods

2 ounces bean pods in $1\frac{1}{2}$ quarts water. Boil for 20 minutes and drink 6 ounces 3 times daily.

Somebody kept from having a cataract operation just by bathing her eyes in warm salt water several times a day. The doctor who had diagnosed cataracts was amazed to examine her later and said, "Why, the Lord gave you your second eyesight!"

CATARRH
Horseradish

1 teaspoon several times.

Catarrhal deafness

Garlic.

CELIAC DISEASE
Banana

Banana is a godsend with celiac. Children are so limited in their food intake, but banana goes well and, by and by, corrects the altered intestinal functions.

CELLULITE
Eggplant

Eggplant has to be sliced and placed in slightly salted water for about 20 minutes or more to remove the bitterness. The skin is extremely helpful. Peel the eggplant $\frac{1}{2}$-inch thick. Boil the peelings until done. Season with kelp or dulse. This is an excellent antidote to tumors and cellulite.

CHICKEN SOUP
Attention

All commercially available meat has to be prepared so the hormones and toxins will be neutralized. Take a chicken or turkey or steak, rub it with plenty of salt, and let it sit for 1 hour. Then rinse it off and prepare it the way you want it. You also can set fowl in buttermilk, which draws the toxins out, especially the feared hormones. Rinse off fowl after soaking it.

Try it! It is delicious, absolutely delicious, like old-fashioned chicken soup.

Why is chicken soup superior to all the things we have, even more relaxing than Tylenol? It is because chicken soup has a natural ingredient which feeds, repairs, and calms the mucous lining in the small intestine. This inner lining is the beginning or ending of the nervous system. It is easily pulled away from the intestine by too many laxatives, too many food additives (chemicals), the wrong food combinations, and parasites. Chicken soup, prepared the above way, heals the nerves, improves digestion, reduces allergies, relaxes, and gives strength.

CHILDREN, NAUGHTY
Cranberry juice with cloves, cinnamon, honey

(*See* LEAD POISONING)

CHILDREN, TOE-WALKING
Chickpea

CHILDREN WHO DO NOT TALK
Fresh strawberries

CHOLESTEROL
Cranberries
> 2 tablespoons cranberry sauce once daily or 1 cup juice a day.

To dissolve cholesterol deposit
> Alfalfa sprouts are best.

CHROMIUM POISON
Thyme tea
> Thyme tea is an antidote to chromium poison which settles in the brain.

CIRCULATION
Cardiac cocktail
> 1 tablespoon paprika, 1 tablespoon vinegar. Gradually substitute cayenne in place of paprika as soon as you can tolerate it. For serious cases take 1 cup of this in warm water 2 times per day.

CIRCULATION TO UTERUS
Tansy

COLDS
Boil in apple juice: cloves, cinnamon, sage, and bay leaves.

Kale
> Gives resistance to colds, has natural sulfur and lots of vitamins.

Onions, white and red
> Make a soup from raw onions, season with Tamari or other broth, and eat.

Broccoli
> Broccoli has natural sulfur which strengthens your resistance to colds.
>
> A, C, iodine, calcium, and trace minerals from elder flower and peppermint.

Thyme
> For resistance to colds or prevention of colds, take thyme tea (1 cup a day).

Grapefruit
> Grate the skin of a grapefruit very finely. Add the juice of 1/2 grapefruit and fill cup with hot water. Grapefruit contains a substance similar to quinine.

Indian remedy
> For chest cold, mix turpentine and coconut butter to a paste, rub on hot wool cloth, and apply to chest or back.

COLITIS
Charcoal

Wild blackberry or red oak bark tea

Creamed papaya

Flax seed tea
> Soak flax seed in plenty of water overnight, bring to a boil, and simmer for 5 minutes. Drink 3 to 4 times a day.

Bananas
> Bananas are excellent to eat when colitis has hit.

Carrot
> Boil carrots until done, blend them or mash then, and eat them. Also drink 6 to 7 ounces of carrot juice 2 times daily.

Spastic colon needs calcium.

COLON INFLAMMATION AND IRRITATION

Irish potato peel and flax seed meal

> Boil a handful of potato peelings in plenty of water. Add 1 tablespoon of flax seed meal to 1 quart of potato peel water and drink 1 cup warm during the day until 1 quart is gone. Do this for 10 to 14 days.

Rutabaga

> Rutabaga is excellent for a weak colon. It is food for the friendly bacteria in the colon and strengthens the membranes of the colon. Boil potatoes with rutabagas, mash them, and eat with butter and salt.

COMPLEXION (cleared)

Cucumber

> Cucumber juice with water. Place slices of cucumber over face where needed.

In general

> 16 ounces prune juice, 1 gallon apple juice each day for 3 days.

CONGESTION

> Foot bath with mustard draws blood out of head. For lungs a mustard plaster with whole-wheat flour, also excellent for kidneys.

CONJUNCTIVITIS

> Place raw potatoes on eyes (grated or sliced).

B_2

CONSTIPATION

1 fig and 3 to 5 prunes

> Soak in warm water overnight. Next morning drink the juice and eat the fruit.

Pears

> 2 raw pears at bedtime. No water with it.

Flax seed

> Soak 1 tablespoon flax seed with 1 tablespoon raisins (currants are best) in 1 cup water. Next morning eat it before breakfast. Mix and soak flax seed with prune juice. Take 1 or 2 tablespoons daily.

Squash with caraway and cream

Figs

    Take 4 white figs, soak them in 1 glass water. Next morning eat the figs and drink the water.

Raw apple

    At bedtime chew an apple very carefully and drink a glass of water with it.

CORNS AND CALLUSES

Corns on feet, sensitive

    Ranunculus = buttercup.

White cabbage

    Grate white cabbage. Add hot water so it is comfortable to your feet. Soak in it for 10 to 20 minutes.

Lemon

    Soak your feet in warm water for about 15 minutes; then cut a small piece of lemon peel and place the inside of it against the corn, tying it on, and let it stay there all night. Do this for 3 nights and the corn should lift out.

COUGH, DRY

Potato peelings

    Boil potato peelings. Sweeten with honey. Take 1 tablespoon several times a day.

Onion

    Boil cut onions in apple cider vinegar. Add honey. 1 teaspoon every hour.

COUGH, PHLEGM

    Ginger tea several times—6 ounces.

COUGH SYRUP

    In 1 cup honey mix 4 drops oil of eucalyptus. Take 1 teaspoon as needed.

Dates, figs, sage

    1 pound dates, 1 pound figs, 1 ounce sage, 4 quarts distilled water. Boil all ingredients for $\frac{1}{2}$ hour, strain, and boil this syrup down to 1 quart. Take this as you need it.

Onion syrup
> Take a yellow onion and make a hole in it. Fill hole with honey or raw sugar. Set it in a saucer and after an hour brown tasty syrup drops out. This is an excellent cough remedy for children and adults.

Honey
> Mix $\frac{1}{2}$ honey and $\frac{1}{2}$ lemon juice.

Cough in children (cramping)
> Boil bread in milk. Make a poultice over throat.

CRIPPLED HANDS
> Mix 1 part sassafras oil with 3 parts almond oil. Massage this mixture daily into hands.

D

DANDRUFF
White beets
> Cut white beets and boil in water until water is almost gone. Strain and take this water to moisten the scalp for 2 to 3 weeks.

Coconut oil
> Secure a small amount of pure coconut oil; rub this in your hair for a few days and dandruff should disappear.

In an old herb book I read:
> Boil a handful of willow leaves. Strain and wash your hair and scalp in it. Put a little concoction aside and dampen the scalp a little every day. I was amazed at the result.

DEBILITY
Ginger tea

DEBILITY OF LIMBS
Daisy tea

DEEP AFFLICTIONS
Tomato

As poultices in deep rooted afflictions. When stewed, good for liver. Fresh tomatoes are a vitamin C supplier. Green tomatoes in very small quantities are a gland stimulant. Always remove the core and stem. Make a deep insertion. This stem part is poisonous.

DEODORIZER
Parsley

Eat some parsley after onions or garlic.

Zinc

Chlorophyll

Everything that is green has chlorophyll. Take plenty of green drinks or buy liquid chlorophyll to combat body odor.

DEPRESSION
Two-thirds of all mental cases are kidney cases.

Juice of 1 pomegranate in the morning, 1 persimmon at noon, and 1 wineglass full of grapefruit juice in the evening keeps you in good humor.

Daisy tea

DETOXIFYING DIET
Seneca Indian Cleansing Diet

This diet was contributed by the Seneca Indians.

First day: Eat only fruits and all you want. Try apples, berries, watermelon, pears, peaches, cherries, whole citrus fruits, and so forth. No bananas.

Second day: Drink all the herb teas you want, such as raspberry, hyssop, chamomile, or peppermint. You may sweeten the tea slightly with honey or maple sugar.

Third day: Eat all the vegetables you want. Have them raw, steamed, or both.

Fourth day: Make a big pot of vegetable broth by boiling cauliflower, cabbage, onion, green pepper, parsley, or whatever you have available. Season with sea salt or vegetable broth cubes. Drink only this rich mineral broth all day long.

This diet has the following effect: The first day the colon (your wastebasket) is cleansed. The second day you release toxins, salt, and excessive calcium deposits in the muscles, tissues, and organs. The third day the digestive tract is supplied with healthful, mineral rich bulk. On the fourth day the blood, lymph, and inner organs are mineralized. That makes a lot of sense!

DE-WORMER
Figs or pomegranate

DIABETES
2 raw string beans daily, Jerusalem artichoke, parsley leaves.

Watercress

Watercress is extra good for the diabetic. Make a big salad out of one bunch of watercress for lunch. Since this is not always available, eat when you have it.

Paprika (zinc) will save eyesight in diabetics.

DIAPER RASH

We have found that vitamin A and D ointment is the best remedy! Be sure to dry the diapers in the sunlight after washing them.

DIARRHEA
Colon food

Blackberries

Blackberries as a juice or as wine, Dr. Houston says, is a remarkable remedy for diarrhea.

Rice gruel

Ripe, raw grated apples

Black pepper

Black pepper as a tea for running bowels.

Arrowroot starch

Take 1 teaspoon arrowroot. Make a paste with water and stir into 7 ounces boiling water, add applesauce to taste.

Black tea

1 or 2 cups without sugar, sipped slowly.

Iceberg lettuce
   Iceberg lettuce has a natural opium which is terribly constipating.

DIGESTION
Flax seed
   Flax seed tea is so soothing to an irritated digestive tract. It coats
   and heals and nourishes. Take 2 tablespoons of flax seed to
   1 quart of water. Simmer for 20 minutes, strain, and drink 1 cup
   of the warm mixture every 2 hours. For best results alternate
   with carrot juice, 1 hour carrot juice, the next hour flax seed tea.

DIGESTION IMPROVED
Alfalfa seed
   Improves digestion, use it as a tea after meals. 1 teaspoon alfalfa
   seed to 1 cup cold water, bring to a boil, and turn the heat off.
   Let sit for 3 to 5 minutes.

DIGESTION WEAK
Zucchini
   Wash zucchini and cut into pieces. Steam or boil with little water,
   place on plate, and sprinkle with ground almonds.

DIGESTIVE HELP
Arrowroot
   It is a food for the weak, debilitated, and those who are conva-
   lescing. Very easily digestible, creating no gastric upset, it forms
   a nourishing diet. People suffering from bacillary dysentery and
   gastric upset would find it most suitable. Take a spoonful of
   arrowroot, make a smooth paste with cold milk or water, stir
   well, and boil. Add a little lime juice before taking it.

DIGESTIVE PROBLEMS
Skin of fruits
   Peel pears, apples, pineapples, peaches, apricots, some of each
   or whatever you have. Take the peelings and simmer 3 to 5 minutes in plenty of water, drink 7 ounces several times a day.

DIGESTIVE PROBLEMS IN CHILDREN
Apple concentrate
   2 teaspoons concentrate in water before meals.

DIURETICS
For kidney stones

Use cucumber juice or tea from $1/2$ avocado leaf. Or take 3 teaspoons of brown corn seed and put in 1 pint of water. Allow to steep, then drink 1 cup daily. This is said also to be good for gallstones.

Cucumber

Cucumber is a very good diuretic. Cucumber contains a hormone needed by the pancreas to produce insulin. It is a specific for skin troubles.

Seeds

Take equal parts of caraway, fennel, and anise, 1 teaspoon each for 1 cup.

DIZZINESS

Rinse mouth with 1 tablespoon of apple cider vinegar.

DIZZINESS WITH DEAFNESS

Take 1 teaspoon horseradish every morning.

DNA

Repaired and strengthened by folic acid.

DOUCHE

1 pint apple brandy, 1 teaspoon sea salt. Shake. Use 2 tablespoons to 1 quart water. Excellent.

DROPSY

$1/2$ gallon apple cider; 1 handful parsley, crushed; 1 handful horseradish, crushed; 1 tablespoon juniper berries. Put in cider, let stand 24 hours in a warm place before use. Take $1/2$ glass 3 times per day before meals.

Horseradish in apple juice

Take $1/2$ cup 3 times a day.

DRUG ADDICTION
Epsom salts

Place 3 to 5 pounds of Epsom salts in a tub of hot water, let person soak for 20 minutes.

From Denmark
>Boil equal parts of carrots, onions, potatoes, celeriac (celery root). Take once a day for 7 days. Add salt and butter.

DRUG RESIDUE
Lima beans
>Make a healthful dish of lima beans, bell peppers, and sweet potatoes. Eat this once a day for 7 days.

DULL PAIN (under both shoulder blades)
Kelp

Baking soda
>Rub on painful area.

(*See also* SHOULDER PAIN)

E

EAR NOISES
Onion juice or cabbage juice
>Drop 1 or 2 drops of onion juice into the ear.

>You may also try cabbage juice mixed with honey, 1 or 2 drops in the ear for lost hearing.

Watercress, figs, and mustard
>Cut and mash and make a poultice over the ear.

EARACHE
Black pepper
>Oil a piece of cotton and sprinkle it with black pepper. Place it over the ear, not in the ear canal.

>Rub oil of sassafras around ear, not inside.

EARS
Frozen
>Apply peppermint oil.

EDEMA OF LOWER EYELIDS
Garden radish
> Eat 1 before each meal.

ENDOMETRIOSIS
Tumors all through the uterine wall
> Dr. Carlton Fredericks said "Absolutely *no* carbohydrates—not even bananas." 1000 mg choline with each meal. 500 mg inositol with each meal. Stress B with C, 6 a day. Douche with alum root for bleeding. In 10 days pain will leave. Keep up for 6 weeks.

ENERGY
Grapes
> Grapes give a lot of energy.

Blackstrap molasses
> Provides minerals and iron.

Flax seed
> $1/2$ tablespoon flax seed, steep in $1/2$ pint hot water. Drink 2 times daily.

ENVIRONMENTAL POISONS (fallout)
Willow leaves

Cinnamon
> Cinnamon removes fallout. Toast 1 slice of bread very brown. Butter it. Sprinkle with cinnamon.

(*See also* FALLOUT)

ENZYME SUPPLIER
Pineapple

EQUILIBRIUM RESTORED
Peppermint
> Rub on back of neck.

EUSTACHIAN TUBE (specific)
Catarrh
> Rose petals.

Stuffed
> Cayenne pepper.

EXHAUSTION
Whey powder
> 1 tablespoon 2 times daily.

EYELIDS
Swollen
> Primrose.
> Put well-beaten egg whites over closed eyes.

Chronic infection
> A, B-complex, C, calcium.

Glued in the morning
> A.

Inflamed
> Apply castor oil.

Stuck in the morning
> Calcium fluoride.

EYES
Burning
> B_2, eyebright.

Infected
> Apply the green leaves of a white lily over the closed eye.

Pinkeye
> Raw grated potatoes over the closed eye. You may also take thin slices of raw potato and cover eye. It will release pain and the redness will go away. Red potatoes are best.

Eye cataract
> Bean pods: 2 ounces bean pods in $1\frac{1}{2}$ quarts water, boil for 20 minutes, and drink 6 ounces 3 times daily.

Eye food
> Sunflower seeds: $\frac{1}{2}$ cup daily.
> Carrot juice: 8 ounces 2 times daily.

Eye pains
> Raw potato: poultice over eye.

Eye problems
> Raw red potatoes: grate 1 raw potato and use as a poultice over the eyes for 1 hour every day. Will improve eye conditions. Even cataracts have been known to be greatly benefited.

EYES AND DIGESTION (increases pepsin)
Bell pepper

EYES, BLOOD AND LYMPH
Carrots

EYES, TIRED
> Dr. Hohensee promoted the following formula for the eyes: Juices of $\frac{1}{2}$ potato, $\frac{1}{2}$ onion, and $\frac{1}{4}$ green pepper. Drink 8 ounces of this $\frac{1}{2}$ hour before your supper and watch your eyes get clearer after 30 days.

Red potatoes
> Raw poultices.

EYESTRAIN
Sunflower seeds
> Nibble about $\frac{1}{2}$ cup of sunflower seeds daily, just 1 or 2 teaspoons will not do.

F

FALLOUT
Cinnamon

> Cinnamon removes fallout. Toast one slice of bread very brown. Butter it and put cinnamon on it. If you like you may also use some brown sugar. This counteracts radiation.

Cloves

> Cloves boiled in cranberry juice and willow leaves in bath water or as a tea.

Soda, salt

> 1 tablespoon soda (baking), 1 tablespoon salt in a tub of warm water. Soak for 15 to 20 minutes, wash or shower with fresh water.

Soda, borax

> 3 tablespoons baking soda, 1 tablespoon borax. Mix and take $^{1}/_{2}$ teaspoon before meals.

(*See also* ENVIRONMENTAL POISONS)

FAT DEPOSITS
Carrot juice

> Carrot juice is believed to be the most perfectly balanced juice available today. It not only readily gives up its energy to the body but, through its vitamin and mineral content, helps the body to release energy from the fat stores. Like green drink, however, it does not store well and should be made up fresh and drunk immediately if possible.

FEAR OF EXAMINATION
Cashew nut

FEELING TOO ...

Cold

Seaweed

Kelp

Cayenne (in hot water)

Hot

Motherwort

FEET ACHING

Hot pepper

If hot peppers upset your stomach, sprinkle hot peppers on the soles of your feet and put on your socks. Hot peppers and radishes contain benzene which is needed for proper functioning of feet and sinuses.

FEET BURNING

Tomato

Try tomato slices on the soles of your feet.

FEET, FEELING OF DEADNESS

Bathe in potato water.

FEET PAINFUL

Lemon juice

Soothe sensitive feet. If the soles of your feet look red and irritated, you might try this simple home remedy. Add 3 teaspoons of lemon juice (or vinegar or boric acid) to 1 quart of water. Rinse your feet in this solution 2 times a day. It is supposed to help soothe and refresh sensitive skin.

FEET SWOLLEN

When feet are swollen in the morning

Male fern root: boil 2 ounces fern in 3 quarts water for 30 minutes. Strain and let cool so it is comfortable to your feet. Bathe feet in it. Save the liquid for the next day.

When feet are swollen at night

Vinegar water compresses.

FEMALE BLEEDING

Okra

2 tablespoons cooked okra 3 times a day will regulate female bleeding. You may ask for *Okra Tablets* in your health food store.

FEMALE COMPLAINTS
Okra

(*See* FEMALE BLEEDING)

FEVER
In all fever diseases there should be a fasting period of 2 days. The patient should have plenty of liquids, such as:

> diluted apple juice
> diluted grape juice
> herb tea with honey
> cherry juice
> fresh orange juice
> lime and lemonade

Herbal
> Black pepper.

Spice tea
> Use equal parts of cardamom and cloves.

FEVER AND FLU
Onion
> Make an onion soup. This soup will bring vitamin C to work.

FEVERISH FEELING
Ginger, black pepper, and honey

(*See also* HEADACHE)

FINGERNAIL CHEWER
Lack of calcium
> Calcium rich foods are carrots and cauliflower.

FLATULENCE
Dill, anise, star anise
> Equal parts, make tea.

FLATUS
Allspice

FLU DESTROYER
Grapefruit
> Freshly squeezed grapefruit diluted with water. Equal parts water and grapefruit juice will ease the flu.

Lettuce leaves
> Take leaf lettuce and boil it in plenty of water. Drink 6 ounces every hour.

FOOD PERFECT
Indian corn

FOOD POISONING
Vinegar
> Take 2 teaspoons apple cider vinegar in 1 glass water (no honey) and sip—drink this. Repeat every hour until all signs of food poisoning are gone.

In case of severe vomiting
> Moisten a cloth with warm vinegar and apply to abdomen.

FOOT CRAMPS
Sulfur
> Put sulfur or cayenne pepper in your socks.

FORGETFULNESS
Sage tea
> 2 cups a day

Mustard seeds

FRECKLES
Lemon
> Rub stain with a few drops of lemon.

FROSTBITE
Lentils
> As compress.

FUNGUS
Fungus grows in alkaline medium. Natural antibiotics are: grapefruit, garlic, willow, radish, chlorophyll, and bee pollen.

Asparagus
> 2 tablespoons 2 times daily.

Concord grape juice
> 3 glasses daily.

G

GALL BLADDER

Lemon juice

> Fresh lemon juice in 1 cup of hot water taken first thing in the morning will empty your gall bladder and start the day on a happy schedule.

> Two teaspoons lemon juice before each meal will strengthen the gall bladder.

Radishes

> Insufficient bile output can be aided by eating one small red radish (or white) before each meal.

Pumpkin seeds

> Take 1 heaping teaspoon ground pumpkin seeds. Put 7 ounces hot water over it and drink it slowly. 2 cups a day are needed.

Horseradish

> Horseradish raw or dried will aid gall bladder.

GALLSTONES

First day:

8 A.M.	1 glass	(8 oz.)	apple juice
10 A.M.	2 glasses	(16 oz.)	apple juice
12 P.M.	2 glasses	(16 oz.)	apple juice
2 P.M.	2 glasses	(16 oz.)	apple juice
4 P.M.	2 glasses	(16 oz.)	apple juice
6 P.M.	2 glasses	(16 oz.)	apple juice

(Juice should be natural, without chemicals.)

Second day:

> Same procedure as the first day. No food. At bedtime 4 ounces olive oil. You may wash the olive oil down with hot lemon juice.

Black radish, olive oil

> Take 2 tablespoons grated black radish blended with 1 tablespoon olive oil. Take 20 minutes before meals for gallstones.

GANGRENE
Tomatoes

> Raw mashed tomatoes every 2 hours over the gangrene, then 1 hour rest. Leave on all night.

Tobacco leaves

> Poultice of tobacco leaves crushed (heals in 10 days).

GASTRIC ULCER
Cabbage

> Scientific research has proven that the juice of raw cabbage is very useful for gastric ulcers because it contains vitamin U.

Cabbage juice

> Freshly made cabbage juice, 6 ounces before meals.

Potato juice

> Freshly made potato juice, 7 ounces between meals.

Carrots

> Nothing to eat but cooked carrots for 7 days.

Potato soup made with milk

GASTRIC UPSET
Arrowroot

> Take a teaspoonful of arrowroot, make a smooth paste with cold milk or water, stir well, and boil. Add a little lime juice just before taking it.

GLAND FOOD
Avocado

> Serve without oil and butter.

Sesame seeds

Sunflower seeds

Sweet potatoes

Yams

GLAND SWELLING
Watercress

> Juice—1 tablespoon 5 times daily.
> Salad—eaten with a slice of buttered bread.

GLAND SWELLING IN NECK
Yellow onion, banana
> Bake yellow onion in oven until done. Mash and apply to throat as a poultice, or bake a banana and do the same.

GLAUCOMA
Yellow onion
> Take a thin slice of yellow onion and hold over closed eyes. When tears come, take onion away and wash eyes in fresh cold water. Do this every day for several weeks.

> No sugar of any kind if you have glaucoma.

GOITER
Agar-agar
> 1 teaspoon 2 times a day. Also cool compresses overnight.

GOOD HEALTH
Dates and milk

GOUT
Onion
> Make raw onion poultice over afflicted area. Leave it on all night.

GOUT AND STONE REMEDY
1 quart apple cider, 1 teaspoon hydrangea root
> Let these stand for 12 hours, bring to a boil, simmer. Take ½ cup 3 times daily.

Sour cherries
> Take 1 small dish of sour cherries every morning for 3 weeks.

GREYING OF HAIR
Sage tea
> Drink and apply.

Nettle tea
> Drink and apply.

GUMS

Epsom salts

Hold a weak solution of Epsom salts in your mouth.

Parsley tea

Use as a wash.

(*See also* BLEEDING GUMS)

H

HALITOSIS

(*See* MOUTH ODOR)

HALLUCINATION

Anacardium occidentale (cashew nut)

Nights

Valerian root

HAY FEVER

Carrots

Cut 3 carrots and cover with 1 quart water and boil for 20 minutes. Drink this broth as an exchange for the vegetable broth suggested.

Vegetable broth

Every half hour drink 4 ounces of pure water. Do this for 2 days. Then make yourself a vegetable broth and drink on the full hour 6 ounces of broth and on the half hour 4 ounces of water.

HEADACHE

Radiating from one point

Black tea, 1 cup.

Vinegar

>Wet a handkerchief with half and half vinegar and water. Place over forehead. Also good for feverish condition.

If headache starts at top of head, it points to intestinal trouble. If it starts at forehead, it is kidney trouble. If it starts at back of head, it is liver and gall bladder trouble.

HEARING, LOSS OF

Horseradish

>2 drops of fresh horseradish juice in each ear.

HEART ATTACK

>Compresses to the heart with vinegar water until physician arrives.

HEART CRAMP

Fennel

>Fennel seed or anise as a tea.

HEART, FIBRILLATION

>Rosemary tea; chew on basil herb; lemon juice with cloves.

HEART, GENERAL

Olive

>Olives are rich in potassium. Soak them and add the brew to your homemade potassium broth.
>
>E, B-complex, C, magnesium, calcium, lecithin.

Specific

>Cramps at night: calcium
>Enlarged: B_1, asparagus
>Extra beats: B_1
>Too fast: B_1
>Nervous palpitation: B-complex, B_6, lecithin, magnesium, calcium, and trace minerals from valerian root.
>Palpitation at night: calcium
>Heart and chest pressure: iodine
>Heart food: the best—*Heartwarmer*
>Muscle: rosemary, hawthorn
>Valves: *Blue Malva Tea*

HEART PAIN
Irregularity

> Chew basil or cinnamon pieces; rosemary tea; lemon water with cloves. See your physician.

> Biotin.

HEART, PALPITATION

> Chew on a piece of cinnamon.

HEART TONIC

> To restore electrical part of heart: 4 tablespoons cane sugar, 4 tablespoons beet sugar, 4 tablespoons corn sugar, 2 teaspoons kosher or sea salt, and 2 teaspoons baking soda. Take 1 teaspoon 2 to 3 times daily.

HEART WEAKNESS
Slow pulse

> Take 1 quart water, add 2 tablespoons vinegar. Wet a small towel and apply over chest close to the heart. Cover with woolen cloth. Change every hour. Results after several hours.

Old recipe

> The following recipe comes from the great mystic of the Middle Ages, Hildegard von Bingen. Her knowledge of herbs was hidden for many years. It is through the work of Dr. G. Hertzka that this writing has come to light.

> Take 10 long stemmed parsley, cut into ¹/₂-inch pieces (leaves and stems are used), and cover with 1 quart natural white wine. Add 1 tablespoon apple cider vinegar and bring to a boil. Simmer for 10 minutes and then add ³/₄ cup of good honey. Now boil again for another 5 minutes. Strain the wine and pour into hot sterile bottles. Close bottles tightly or set in the refrigerator. Caution: wine will run over easily while heating, so stay with it.

> Whenever you feel weakness or aches around the heart or you are overworked, take 3 tablespoons of this tonic 2 to 3 times daily. Parsley wine strengthens heart nerves and heart muscle and your heart's entire function becomes stabilized.

HEARTBURN
Potato

> Eat a slice of raw potato when you have heartburn.

HEAVINESS
Stomach
> Ginger tea.

Eyelids
> Violet leaves.

HEMORRHAGE FROM BLADDER
Peach
> Peach tree bark as a tea. Also magnesium.

HEMORRHOIDS
Potato
> Out of a piece of raw potato form a suppository. At night put into rectum.

Almonds
> Eat 3 almonds a day to prevent and eliminate hemorrhoids.

Garlic
> Take a clove of garlic. Oil it and insert it into the rectum each night for several nights in a row.

Sage
> Make a little pillow, fill with sage leaves, and keep it in place overnight—safety pin it in place to your underwear.

HEROIN DEPOSITS
> Chaparral or bathe in tobacco water.

HICCUPS
> Blow into a paper bag.

Vinegar
> A few drops of vinegar on 1 teaspoon of sugar.
> 1 spoonful of vinegar in some water.

Anise
> Make one cup of anise tea and sip slowly.

Pineapple juice
> Pineapple juice relieves hiccups.

HOARSENESS
Ginger tea

Black bean juice
>Take black beans and boil them in plenty of water, 1 pound of beans to 1 gallon water. Boil for 1 hour, strain. Drink the juice, 6 ounces 3 to 4 times daily. Eat beans in another dish or in soup.

Glycerin
>1 tablespoon glycerin in hot water, gargle often.

HOMESICKNESS
Cayenne pepper

HOOKWORM
Thyme tea
>2 cups strong thyme tea followed by a dose of Epsom salts. Take Epsom salts ½ hour after the thyme tea.

HORMONE, FEMALE
Black cohosh, rice polishings

Booster
>½ cup ground cashews, 2 tablespoons rice polishings, 2 cups water or apple juice. Blend in blender, add honey if wanted. This gives women charm and femininity.

Supply
>Pumpkin seeds.

HORMONE, MALE
Sarsaparilla, brewer's yeast

Booster
>2 tablespoons brewer's yeast, 1 teaspoon chia seed, 1 cup cashews, 2 cups tomato juice, blend in blender. This will give men will power and determination.

Supply
>Pumpkin seeds.

HUNGRY, BUT FEELING FULL AFTER A FEW BITES
Choline

HYPERTENSION
Onions

Chemists found that onions contain a substance called prosta-glandin. This is normally produced in the human body and is known to have an anti-hypertensive effect.

HYPOCHONDRIA
Vanilla

Take 1 vanilla bean, cut in pieces. Boil it in 1 cup of water for 5 minutes. Sweeten with honey.

Cherries

Eat cherries morning and night for hypochondria.

HYPOGLYCEMIA

3 drops oil of sassafras in 1 tablespoon fruit juice 2 times daily for 4 weeks.

I

INDIGESTION
Summer savory

Citrus family
> To 1 quart water add the juice of 1 grapefruit, 1 lemon, 3 oranges, 2 tablespoons milk sugar, 1 cup aloe vera. Drink in small sips 1 quart per day.

Whey
> 1 tablespoon of whey in a little water will help digestion.

INFANT COLIC
Caraway and anise seed tea

INFECTIONS
The natural antibiotics are:
> Garlic
> Grapefruit
> Chlorophyll
> Parsley and radish
> Willow
> Bee pollen extract

Cranberries
> Boil cranberries and use the juice.

Potato
> Suck raw potatoes and spit out the pulp. Or make 1 cup raw potato juice, add to 3 cups water, and drink.

Infectious diseases
> Compresses of warm milk all over the body. Wrap patient in first layer of warm milk sheet, second layer woolen blanket, and third layer warm cover. In 2 hours repeat if needed.

In sinus
> Pepper and honey. Take 1 teaspoon honey and sprinkle with freshly ground pepper. Eat it. Also good for sniffles.

Staph
> Grapefruit. Grate the skin of a grapefruit with a fine grater. Take 1 teaspoon and add the juice of 1/2 grapefruit. Drink this 3 times a day.

In lung
> Onion. Boil onions, mash them, and place them between 2 layers of cloth. Apply to chest for about 2 hours.

Infectious hepatitis
> Calendula (marigold).
> Fresh lime juice.

Skin
> White pond lily.

INFLAMMATIONS
Inflammation of the colon
> Irish potato peel and flax seed meal. Make tea.

Inflammation of eye and eyelid
> Elder flower (externally). Also drink 2 cups a day. Raw potato poultice over eye.

Inflamed nerves
> Peppermint tea, peppermint lotion.

INNER EAR
Horsetail bath

Sassafras oil around ear, not inside.

INSECT BITES
Sage tea
> Rub it on

Plantain leaf

Yellow onion

Bee sting
> On tongue, 1 teaspoon salt. Has helped many from suffocating.

(*See also* BEE STING)

Apple
> Place a piece of raw apple on the bite.

Vinegar
> Mix vinegar with flax and apply.

(*See also* MOSQUITO BITE)

INSECT REPELLENT
> Rub parsley tea on skin.

INSOMNIA
From gas
> 10 drops of eucalyptus oil at bedtime in capsules.

Squaw vine

Oats
> Boil whole grain oats in plenty of water. Strain the oats and season the water with lemon juice and honey. Oats should have the husks on because the healing part is found in the hulls and husks.

INSULIN PRODUCER
Cucumber
> Cucumber contains a hormone needed to produce insulin.

INTERFERON
Cottage cheese
> Cottage cheese is very valuable and I share with you the recipe of Dr. H. Budwig. With the following recipe the body makes its own interferon.
>
> FOUNDATION RECIPE: Put in blender or mix thoroughly by hand: 1 cup cottage cheese and 2 tablespoons walnut or almond oil. This mixture is the foundation recipe and can be varied.
>
> A. To foundation recipe add finely grated horseradish. Serve with potatoes, buckwheat, and/or stewed carrots.
>
> B. To foundation recipe add spices such as finely cut parsley, celery, or paprika.

C. To foundation recipe add tomatoes or tomato puree to taste. This is very delicious with rice, bulgur, or rye bread.

D. To foundation recipe add chives, onion, parsley (finely cut), or paprika.

E. Make a colorful surprise by adding color: To one part of the cottage cheese add tomato puree or beets; to second part add greens such as spinach; to third part add egg yolk. Arrange nicely and decorate with cucumber, tomatoes, radishes, etc.

F. Heap the foundation recipe on lettuce leaves.

G. As a dessert, sweeten the foundation recipe with honey. Add a banana, a grated apple, and some oat flakes on top.

H. To cottage cheese mixture add honey, filberts, almonds, all finely cut. Do not use peanuts. This is terrific for the center of a variety fruit plate. It is a whole meal!

INTESTINAL DIFFICULTIES
Potato drink
> Boil 2 medium potatoes, cut in pieces in 1 quart water, with peeling; pour 4 cups of potato water over 3 tablespoons flax seed (ground) and 6 tablespoons bran. Let stand overnight with lemon or orange juice and a small, finely chopped onion. It tastes good and is more nutritious.

Intestinal catarrh
> Ginger tea.

Intestinal disorder
> 1 cup aloe vera juice, 1 quart water, juice of 1 grapefruit, 3 oranges, 1 lemon, 3 tablespoons milk sugar, and honey to taste.
> Or honey to taste, 1 grapefruit, 1 lemon, 3 tablespoons milk sugar, 1/2 cup aloe vera juice.

Intestinal mucous
> Garlic.

INTESTINES GRIPPING
Coriander

INTOXICATION
> Honey removes alcohol from the blood extra fast.

(*See also* ALCOHOL)

48

IODINE SUPPLIER
Fish

ITCHY SKIN
Marjoram

J

JAUNDICE
Lime

When one has jaundice due to infection or hepatitis, buy the fruit known as limes and make yourself fresh lime water. Sweeten it with honey. This is all you get. Drink 6 to 8 ounces of this refreshing drink every hour. Soon your appetite will come back and you will think of all the goodies a pastry shop has to offer. Do not be tempted! Stick with the juice until you are dreadfully hungry. This might take about 2 to 3 days. Then break the juice diet with a small dish of cooked beets and/or cooked carrots. If you tolerate this well, you may add, 4 hours later, a piece of baked potato without butter or sour cream. Always drink the lime water. Next day add a little fat free yogurt or cottage cheese and some well-done rice. In one week's time, you should be back on your feet.

JOINTS
Swollen

Extract potato juice and boil down to $^1/_5$. Add glycerin to preserve it. Make poultice.

Lubricate

Here is a marvelous recipe to lubricate joints and make joints supple. A young girl, a flower child, gave it to me. I wish I could show to everyone the lovely drawing she put under the recipe.

1 teaspoon turmeric
2 teaspoons almond oil
2 tablespoons soy milk powder
1 cup water
salt and honey to taste

Heat this and serve as a lovely hot drink.

Joint pains
> Simmer laurel beans in any oil and apply over aching joints.

Joints feel weak
> Ginger tea.

Joint trouble
> Sulfur.

K

KIDNEY AND/OR BLADDER STONES
Parsley
> Drink parsley tea for 3 days with no other food.

Asparagus
> Asparagus dissolves oxalic acid crystals when they are lodged in the kidneys.

Grape juice
> Take 1 cup or 7 ounces of dark grape juice, add $\frac{1}{2}$ teaspoon cream of tartar. Take 2 ounces 3 times daily before meals.

Dandelion root
> Boil in apple juice for kidney stones. 2 tablespoons dandelion root to 1 quart water.

Beets
> Boil 5 whole medium sized beets in 3 quarts of water for 1 hour. Drink 7 ounces of the water 3 times daily.

Diuretic for kidney stones
> Use cucumber juice or tea from $\frac{1}{2}$ avocado leaf. Or take brown corn water—allow to steep, then drink 1 cup daily.

KIDNEY DYSFUNCTION
Asparagus

Asparagus is strongly diuretic in action. Boil asparagus in plenty of water and use the concoction 1 cup 4 times daily. 2 quarts water to 4 ounces asparagus.

KIDNEY INFECTION
Watermelon

All the watermelon you want for 2 days, no other food.

KIDNEY INFLAMMATION (Bright's disease)
Watermelon and its seeds

For 2 days, eat nothing but watermelon. Always eat watermelon by itself.

Indian remedy

One radish 3 times a day.

KIDNEY PROBLEMS
Celery tops

For kidney and bladder troubles, eat celery tops after each meal for 5 weeks.

KIDNEY TROUBLE
Cranberry juice

$^1/_2$ cranberry juice, $^1/_2$ water. Take 7 ounces 3 times daily.

KNEES KNOCK AGAINST EACH OTHER
Lathyrus sativus (chickpea)

KNEES SWOLLEN
Cabbage

Grate white cabbage and put in cheesecloth. Apply over swollen knee several nights in a row.

L

LARYNGITIS
Black bean

(*See* HOARSENESS)

LARYNX TICKLING
Red onion
>Raw or as soup.

LAXATIVE
Prunes, apricots
>Mix prunes and apricots, 3 apricots and 3 prunes. Soak overnight and take this much 2 times daily. This combination is special.

LEAD POISONING
>1 gallon commercial cranberry juice
>3 tablespoons whole cloves
>2 teaspoons ground cinnamon
>1 teaspoon cream of tartar

>Boil the cloves in 1 quart cranberry juice for 20 minutes. Strain and add 2 teaspoons ground cinnamon. Stir and add to the rest of the cranberry juice. Now add 1 teaspoon cream of tartar, stir. Drink 5 ounces 3 times daily for 12 to 15 days. Then do it once a week. For children, 3 ounces 3 times daily.

Cabbage
>Cabbage counteracts lead poisoning. Cranberries are also helpful.

(*See also* CHILDREN, NAUGHTY)

LEG TROUBLE
Male fern baths

Calcium
>Cramps at night may be lead accumulations.

LEUKEMIA
Sulfur herbs

Red beets
> Red beet has been valued since ancient times because of valuable factors that can contribute substantially to the health of the body.

Okra
> Okra gives strength to one suffering from leukemia

Shortage of zinc
> Chlorophyll from watermelon rind and seeds.

LIVER
Apricots, pineapple juice
> Apricots are a splendid remedy to detoxify the liver and the pancreas. Soak 1 pound dried apricots in pineapple juice. Next morning blend it and juice of fresh pineapples. Take this 2 days in a row.

Casaba melon
> Take a casaba melon by itself.

Carrot juice
> 6 ounces of carrot juice, 2 tablespoons cream taken 1 hour after breakfast.
> $1/2$ quart carrot juice
> $1/2$ quart goat's milk
> 1 tablespoon molasses per quart

LIVER AILMENT
Breakfast
> 2 tablespoons ground flax seed
> 2 tablespoons whey
> 2 peeled and finely grated apples

> Mix and serve with honey. It is nourishing, tasty, and healing to the liver and intestines.

LIVER ENLARGEMENT
Flax seed
> Place flax seed in a little bag, hang it in boiling hot water for 10 minutes, squeeze excess water out, and apply over liver area. Cover with a towel.

LIVER FOOD
Dandelion leaves

LIVER, SWOLLEN
Potato
> Cook red potatoes, mash them, place between two layers of cloth, and apply warm to the liver.

LUNG ABSCESSES
Cucumber juice

LUNG DISEASES
> Add dill to your food. Eat fish, vegetables, salads, very few carbohydrates, and lots of cream, fat, or butter.

LUPUS (skin)
> Bring wine vinegar to a boil and thicken it with barley flour. Apply to skin.

LYMPH CLEANSER
Barley
> Boil 3 tablespoons barley in 1 quart water for 30 minutes. Strain. Add a little clove and cinnamon. Drink this in 1 day. It will clear the congestion in the lymphatic system.

LYMPHATIC SYSTEM
Cucumber
> 4 to 5 cups of cucumber juice a day for 1 week purifies the lymphatic system and the blood and clears the complexion.

M

MALARIA
Collard seed, parsley seed, red pepper seed

MEMORY
Almonds

> An excellent tonic for the brain. Take 6 to 10 a day. Almond oil improves the memory also. Take 1 teaspoon a day.

Sage

> Make a sandwich of sage. 1 slice thickly buttered dark bread, sprinkle generously with sage. Cover it with another thin slice of bread. You have never tasted such a delicacy.

Cloves

> Cloves in your tea will heighten your memory: 4 cloves in any tea mixture.

Mustard seeds

> 2 mustard seeds for memory

Prunes

> To improve your memory take 3 prunes daily.

METALLIC POISON
Green beans, zucchini

> Zucchini and green beans eaten exclusively for 3 days will get rid of metallic poison.

Squash and strawberries

> Remove arsenic poison. Extra good for smokers. It also removes other metallic poisons.

Mexican raw sugar
Take 1 teaspoonful several times a day until symptoms subside.

(*See also* POISON, METALS)

MILK ALLERGY
Parsnip
Boil parsnip in plenty of water. After it is done, blend it to a smooth pulp. Whenever one is sensitive to milk products, give them 1 to 2 teaspoons of parsnip pulp to eat before drinking milk.

MILK LEG
Cayenne externally

MINERAL SUPPLIER
Alfalfa seeds
As sprouts, tea, or tablets.

MORNING SICKNESS
B_6 and trace minerals from peach leaf tea

MORPHINE HABIT
Oats

MOSQUITO BITE
Bar soap
Moisten a little and rub over bite. It will stop itching.

MOTHER'S MILK, DRY UP
Cranesbill
(Strong tea.) Massage into breasts.

Sage tea
3 cups a day.

MOTHER'S MILK INCREASED
Caraway
1 teaspoonful caraway seed in 8 ounces cold water. Bring to a boil, simmer for a few minutes, and drink several cups a day to increase mother's milk.

Fennel seed in barley water

Alfalfa, blessed thistle

Lentils
> Lentils give good, rich milk.

MOUTH, BURNING
> Make a tea of poppy seed (available in your spice section). Hold tea in your mouth several times a day.

MOUTH, DRY
> Chew cloves.

MOUTH ODOR
> Chew juniper berries, caraway seed, or parsley leaves.

MUCOUS
Oranges
> Mucous cleansers of the stomach, ears, head, and sinuses if taken in the following manner:
>
> 1 glass fresh orange juice
> Same amount distilled water
>
> Do not mix. First drink the orange juice, then follow with the water. Do this as often as you want, 10 times a day or so. Do it 2 days in a row 2 to 3 times a year.

MULTIPLE SCLEROSIS
Pineapple and avocado

MUSCLE BUILDERS
Beans and corn
> The combination of beans and corn makes strong muscles, in combinations such as beans and cornbread or corn tortillas and beans.

Rye

MUSCLE PAIN
> Rub a piece of raw potato over the muscle.

MUSCLE STRENGTH
Chia seed
> Soak 1 teaspoon chia seed in 4 ounces of juice for 2 to 3 hours and drink this 3 to 4 times a day.

Buckwheat
> As pancakes, as cereal, or as a main dish.

MUSCLE WEAKNESS
Apple peelings
> Take a handful of apple peelings and boil them for 20 minutes in 1 quart water. Strain and give 6 ounces daily.

Jerusalem artichokes

Sesame seeds
> Complete amino acid supplier. Makes strong-willed people. Supplies osmium, a trace mineral.

MYOPIC ASTIGMATISM
Tiger lily

N

NAUSEA
Summer savory
> If constant ... peach tree bark.

NEPHRITIS
A, B_2

Watermelon seed tea

NERVE FOOD
Pineapple juice, prune juice
> Pineapple juice mixed with prune juice rebuilds exhausted nerves. Take 6 ounces 3 times daily.

Egg yolk
> Two egg yolks from good healthy eggs mixed with 4 ounces grape juice once or twice daily.

Apple whey
> Take 1 pint apple juice or apple wine, 1 pint water, 1 pint milk. Heat it slowly but do not bring to a boil. When it curdles, strain it through a fine cloth. Throw curds away, sweeten with honey if needed. Take 2 tablespoons 5 times daily if person is very weak. Appetite will improve and all signs of illness will disappear. As patient gets stronger, give up to 2 cups a day. It is powerful.

Strawberries
Rich in vitamin C and rich in minerals. Especially good for nervous disorders and to help build up weak kidney and bladder. Eat 4 ounces 2 times daily.

Cherry juice, egg yolk
Add egg yolk to a 6 ounce glass of cherry juice, stir, and drink. It is a wonderful nerve food.

NERVES
Almonds
Blanched almonds with grapes to assist the nerves.

Celery
Eat crisp and tender celery for depleted nerves.

Sage
In bathtub and as tea.

Lavender
In bathtub.

Place a red and green towel in your bed. Sleep on it.

(*See also* SEDATIVE)

NERVOUS DISORDERS
Onion
Onion poultice to calves of legs does wonders.

NEURALGIA
Salt
Heat salt in frying pan or oven. Put in a cloth bag and apply to painful face.

White beet
The leaves and root of the white beet are excellent for neuralgia. Boil and apply to the pain in a small poultice sack.

Mullein oil, yarrow oil, chamomile oil, thyme oil
Mix the oils and apply.

Red onion
As a poultice.

In ankle
    Mullein.

In right ankle
    Yarrow.

In lower jaw
    Prickly ash.
    Raw plantain juice over painful area.

NIGHT SWEATS (profuse)
Dandelion, linden blossom tea

NOISE
Distraction by noise
    B-complex, calcium, magnesium.

NOSE
Polyps
    A strong tea of oak bark, sniffed up the nose several times a day.
    Dulcamera roots made in tea and sniffed several times a day.

Red nose
    Wash with a borax solution and rub strawberries over it.

Dry nose
    Put arms in a warm bath. Add sage to the water. Also boil basil
    in milk and steep a teaspoon of sage in it. Drink 6 ounces a day.
    Sage boiled in milk, 2 tablespoons several times daily.

NUMBNESS IN FINGERTIPS, TONGUE
Chickpea

O

OBESITY
Celery
> A low calorie reducing aid.

Celery seed
> Drink the tea.

OLD AGE
H-12

Primrose flowers

Sauerkraut
> This keeps old age diseases away, such as stiffness, failing eyesight, wrinkles, constipation, and general useless feelings.

OPTIC NERVES
Tomato
> Tomato leaves or peelings—do not boil this, cover leaves with hot water. Let stand 15 minutes, drain, and set in refrigerator. Dosage: 1 teaspoon 3 times daily before meals.

OSMIUM SUPPLIER
Sesame seeds
> Sesame seeds make strong-willed people and prevent nervous breakdown. Also squash, raspberries, and Indian corn are good osmium suppliers.

P

PEP DRINK
Sprouts
> 3 cups pineapple juice
> 1 cup water
> 1 cup alfalfa sprouts
> 10 almonds
>> OR
> 2 cups pineapple juice

Sunflower seeds and dates
> Take 2 tablespoons seeds and dates, blend in blender with 8 to 10 ounces water.

(*See also* BOOSTER)

PEPSIN SUPPLIER
Pineapple juice
> Take 2 ounces pineapple juice before meals.

PERSPIRATION
Linden flower tea, hot lemonade
> To encourage perspiration.

PIMPLES
Nutmeg
> Nutmeg for boils and pimples. Use $1/3$ teaspoon nutmeg (freshly ground), 1 teaspoon honey, and $1/2$ cup hot water. Drink 3 mornings in a row, then 3 mornings not. Repeat this 8 to 9 times.

Epsom salts

> Make a brine of Epsom salts and pat on the face with cotton and let dry before going to bed. Do this until the pimples are dried up.

PINKEYE

Potato

> Raw grated potatoes over the closed eye. You also may take thin slices of raw potato and cover eye. It will release pain and the redness will go away. Red potatoes are best.

PITUITARY

Deficiency

> Cherry bark, cherry juice

Watercress

> Alternate: 1 bunch of watercress a day, next day 6 ounces pineapple juice 2 times daily. Pituitary people have fleshy hands.

PLEURISY

Flax seed

> Flax seed as tea and as poultice.

PNEUMONIA

Collard seeds, parsley seeds, spinach seeds, onion seeds

> Simmer 1 teaspoon of each of the seeds in 1 pint water. 1 pint water needs 4 tablespoons of seeds. Drink 4 ounces every hour.

Milk

> Warm milk compresses around the upper torso. Take a towel, dip in warm milk, wrap around body. Wrap around with plastic, then warm cloth.

> Also—hold right hand over forehead and left hand on lower back of head for 20 minutes.

Cranberry juice

> Give cranberry juice as preferred to any other juice.

POISON IVY

Epsom salts

> Wet Epsom salts and apply to painful area.

Fels Naphtha soap

> Wash with Fels Naphtha soap—no more troubles.

POISON, LEAD

(*See* LEAD POISONING)

POISON, METALS

 2 tablespoons pumpkin seeds, ground
 1 tablespoon okra powder
 $^1/_2$ teaspoon cayenne pepper

When mixed take 1 teaspoon of this in 1 tablespoon rhubarb sauce about 3 times a day for 10 days. One of the most universal remedies to remove lead, arsenic, platinum, gold, and mercury from your body.

(*See also* METALLIC POISON)

POISON OAK

White oak bark
 Tea application.

POISONS, FLUSH

Anise and caraway
 Make a tea and drink 3 cups a day.

POISONS SWALLOWED

Charcoal
 Charcoal will absorb up to $^1/_2$ its weight in poison. Burn a piece of bread, toasting it many times.

PREGNANCY

Peaches
 Peaches are good for pregnant women. It is a complete food for mother and fetus. Also drink peach leaf tea for morning sickness.

Coconut milk
 Pregnant women should take coconut milk regularly in the morning on an empty stomach. It will bring very clear urine and also nourish the fetus, and the child will be a healthy one.

PROTEIN

Avocado
 Don't overlook the avocado as a fat and protein supplier.

Meat
 Meat provides protein that gives an explosive energy. Appetite satisfying.

Lentils
Supply protein and iron of the best quality.

Millet

Meat of the vegetarian, 15 percent protein, millet is easily digested.

PROTEIN DIGESTANT
Celery

Celery aids protein digestion. It increases appetite, is good in curing mucous, and, therefore, is used for rheumatic pain, gastric trouble, cold, cough, and urinary disorders.

PROSTATE
Coconut

The fluid of the coconut (coconut milk) is a specific for toning up the prostate gland.

PROSTATE ENLARGED
Spanish onion juice

Grate a yellow onion, press through a cheesecloth, and take 1 tablespoon 2 times a day.

PROSTATE TROUBLE
Milk

Apply milk compresses as you would diaper a baby. Warm the milk (do not boil), soak a Turkish towel in it, and apply with a hot water bottle.

PUTREFACTION (arrest it)
Charcoal, burnt toast

R

RADIATION
Salt and soda

Add 1 pound baking soda and $\frac{1}{2}$ pound salt to your bath.

Seaweed
> Has neutralizing effect on radiation overdose.

Miso soup
> Also has a neutralizing effect.

RADIOACTIVE FALLOUT

> Radiation cannot be seen or heard. It is a shadow. It is a danger to mankind of immense dimensions. Radiation lingers in the grass that the animals eat. It is in the air and, after rain and snow, we get extra doses of it. It is in the water, it is in all of us.

> 1 teaspoon baking soda
> 1 teaspoon sea salt
> $\frac{1}{2}$ teaspoon cream of tartar
> 1 quart water

> Mix and drink 8 ounces every 2 hours with symptoms leaving with every dose.

Formula from your own kitchen:
> 1 glass cranberry juice
> $\frac{1}{4}$ teaspoon cinnamon
> $\frac{1}{4}$ teaspoon powdered clove
> $\frac{1}{4}$ teaspoon cream of tartar
> This drink is very delicious and helpful.

Willow leaves
> 1 cup of willow leaf tea will help lessen all symptoms of the illness.

RATTLESNAKE BITE
Salt
> Wet some salt and wrap arms or feet in the salt pack. Be sure the bite gets an extra dose of salt. Now rush to your physician.

REDUCING
Dulse, kelp, agar-agar

Leeks
> Cut leeks and boil in water. Use the water and the tougher parts in soup and the tender parts in a salad.

> Leeks are a pancreas food, tissue builder, and brain food.

REJUVENATION
H-12

(*See also* AGING)

REPRODUCTIVE ORGANS
Infection
>Oak bark concoction in bathtub.

Itching of genitals
>Wash with strong sage tea.

RESPIRATORY AILMENT
Celery seeds

RESTLESSNESS
B-complex, B_1, B_6, calcium lactate

Magnesium
>Restless movements of eyes and fingers.

RHEUMATIC FEVER
Apple peeling concentrate

(*See* MUSCLE WEAKNESS)

RHEUMATIC MUSCLES
Asparagus

Sawdust
>Sawdust contains natural DMSO. Take pine sawdust, boil it in water for 10 minutes, and place hands or feet into the warm mush. When in spine, strain mush and place in sack.

Basil
>Eases rheumatism pain. Drink it as a tea and/or sprinkle it on an oiled cloth and apply to aching part.

RHEUMATISM
Rumafix, B-complex, B, B_{15}, C, bioflavonoids, folic acid, calcium
>In many cases but not all.

Chickweed
>If shifting side to side.

Violet root
>In upper part of body, right side.

Basil
>Eases rheumatism pain. Drink it as a tea and/or sprinkle it on an oiled cloth and apply to aching part.

Raw potato

> Carry a raw potato in your pocket. In 1 or 2 days it is all shriveled up and stinks from the poison attracted. Then place another potato in your pocket.

RINGWORM (tinea)
Banana peel

> Rub banana peel on area.

ROUGH SKIN

> Eat silicon rich foods such as oats, wheat bran. Eat oatmeal and rub face and arms with oat water. Wheat bran makes the skin smooth. Make a thin paste of wheat bran and apply to face, neck, and arms.

S

SCAR TISSUE
Cocoa butter

> Rub cocoa butter on scar. It has to be done consistently, 2 times daily.

SEDATIVE (nerve)
Myrtle

(*See also* NERVES)

SENILITY

> Eating food cooked in aluminum pots and pans may cause senility, according to Dr. Stephen E. Levick of Yale. Shocking medical tests reveal that people who are suffering from dementia diseases, exhibiting symptoms similar to senility, have abnormally high concentrations of aluminum in their brains.

SENIOR COLD FEELING
Lemon water with honey and 2 drops of cinnamon oil. Also, boil cinnamon pieces in water for 20 minutes, sweeten with honey.

SHINGLES
Peppermint

Celery
1¹/₂ quarts celery juice daily.

Epsom salts
Make a paste of it by adding water to achieve the right consistency, then apply frequently to the affected parts until relief is felt.

SHOCK
Cayenne pepper in cream

SHORTNESS OF BREATH
Red onion juice
Bring to boil, add honey, simmer for 15 minutes. Take 1 teaspoon every hour.

SHOTS
Suck hard candy for 30 minutes. Spit out all saliva.

SHOULDER PAIN
Dull pains under both shoulder blades
Iodine.

Pain under right shoulder
Gall bladder.

Pain under left shoulder
Stomach.

(*See also* DULL PAIN)

SINUS
Horseradish, onion, turnips, mustard, radishes

Horseradish
Take a piece of fresh horseradish or open a jar of horseradish relish and take a little piece several times a day.

Black pepper
Take 1 teaspoon honey, grind black pepper over it (it must be freshly ground), and take as needed.

SINUS TROUBLE

One tablespoon marjoram with one tablespoon butter, boil 5 minutes and strain through cloth. Rub forehead, nose, cheeks, and nostrils with it.

Sip 12 ounces grape juice 2 times daily for 6 weeks.

SKIN (scaly)
Lecithin

Soybean lecithin for red, itchy, scaly skin. Make a salve and apply it. Also take 2 tablespoons by mouth.

SKIN BLEMISHES
Soda bicarbonate

Make a small paste of spirits of camphor in soda bicarbonate, pat on area involved, and leave on overnight for 1 week. Do not bandage or cover for 1 week.

SKIN PIGMENTATION (dirty, oily, yellowish)
Calcium fluoride

SKIN REMEDY
Cucumber

SKIN TROUBLE
Cucumber

It is a strong diuretic. Cucumber contains a hormone needed by the pancreas to produce insulin. It is a specific for skin troubles.

SKUNK STINK
Tomato juice

Wash body and clothes with ½ cup tomato juice in water and/or ½ cup ammonia in water.

SLEEP WITH EYES HALF OPEN
Magnesium

SLEEPLESSNESS
Magnesium, B, calcium, catnip

Iron
>Sleeplessness at night and sleepy in daytime.

Poppy seeds
>Fill a small sock and lay it on your forehead.

Dill oil
>Rub your forehead with dill oil.

Laurel leaves
>Place in a small bag and lay your head on it.

Anise seed
>Take 1 teaspoon before going to bed.

Honey and milk
>Warm a cup of milk and add 1 teaspoon of honey. Drink before going to bed.

SORES
Honey
>Honey is healing and disinfecting on sores.

SORE THROAT
Ginger
>Chew a piece of ginger or drink ginger tea.

SPASMS DUE TO FALLOUT
Cinnamon on burnt toast

SPEECH, STAGGERS
Nutmeg
>In a small amount of hot water.

SPINAL WEAKNESS
Bran
>Heat bran in your oven, fill up a cloth bag with the warm bran, and apply to spine.

SPLEEN
Eggplant
>It reduces enlarged spleen and increases red blood corpuscles and hemoglobin. Therefore, it is very good for anemia.

SPLEEN FOOD
Pumpkin seeds
> Chew very well.

SPLEEN AND LIVER CLEANSER
> 2 quarts concord grape juice
> juice of 6 oranges
> juice of 3 lemons

> Cut the white of the lemon into small pieces. Boil this in a little water for 10 minutes. Strain. Add the water to the drink. Then take distilled water and fill the liquid mixture to 1 gallon. This is a 1-day supply of your food-drink intake. Just 2 days of this will cleanse your organs, as Drano cleanses your water pipes.

SPLEEN, OBSTRUCTION
Black tea
> 1 cup black tea with a little raw honey will open an obstructed spleen.

SPLINTER
> A splinter in your finger should be removed at once. It if is too deep, apply a fresh piece of onion, tomato, or *Cell Salt No. 12 (Silica)*.

Honey
> Apply honey. Soon the splinter will come to the surface.

Ice cube
> Freeze the area with an ice cube. You can then remove the splinter with no pain.

SPRAINS
> Ice cold water as compress.

Daisy, lavender
> For extra sore sprains, use as compress.

STIES
Black tea
> Make a poultice of black tea, Lipton will do, place moist over the eye, bandage at night.

STIMULANT
Cayenne pepper

STOMACH

The following foods are particularly healing to sick stomachs and ulcers and the pain, discomfort, and suffering from stomach distress. Carrot, coconut milk, eggplant, flax seed tea, okra, parsnip, sweet potato.

Indian remedy

Blackberry wine.

Pepsin

Unsweetened pineapple juice poured over melons develops pepsin which is needed in the stomach for digestion.

Persimmon

Persimmon before meals if stomach does not behave.

Cardamom

Has a soothing effect on all membranes of the stomach and lungs.

Whey

With stomach ailments take 1 tablespoon whey 3 times daily. This will feed the stomach glands and they will work well again.

STOMACH CRAMPS

Apricot brandy

This will stop chronic stomach cramps. Take 1 teaspoon.

STOMACH FLU

Ginger

Use $\frac{1}{2}$ teaspoon ground ginger to 1 cup water. Add 1 teaspoon honey and drink hot. Also, hot compresses of ginger over stomach will bring relief.

STOMACH GAS

Certo, apple juice

1 teaspoon Certo added to $\frac{1}{2}$ glass apple juice, drink as needed.

STOMACH ULCERS

Marigold tea, yarrow tea

Cabbage

Cabbage juice (it must be freshly made) is used for stomach ulcers because of the vitamin U in cabbage.

Okra

Cooked, do not season heavily.

73

Potato

Juice 1 potato, add the same amount of warm water. Drink before each meal, 3 times a day. Red potatoes are best.

Apples

Raw and cooked.

STOMACHACHE

Flax seed

2 teaspoons, cover with 8 ounces boiling water, keep it warm for 30 minutes, and drink 1 to 2 cups.

STOP SMOKING

Calamus root

Chew or cook in apple juice.

(*See also* TOBACCO CRAVING)

STREP INFECTION

Cucumber

Grate cucumber and squeeze the juice out. Drink 5 times a day.

STROKE

Tofu

Shave head, apply tofu over head, and change the compress when tofu gets yellow.

Paralysis after a stroke

Wash the limbs with tobacco water.

Danger of stroke

Rosemary.

Tendency

Sage tea.

Mustard seed

My husband had a partial stroke with paralysis. I gave him a teaspoonful of the whole mustard seed, either black or white will do, every few hours until his face looked flushed.

SUICIDAL
Black tea

Make 2 cups or more black tea, add sugar or honey.

SWELLING
Ankles

Adzuki beans—boil in plenty of water. Eat them as a soup or drink the fluid 2 times a day.

Knees

Raw cabbage is terrific for poultices over swollen knees or elbows. Grate 2 cups of cabbage very fine. Wrap in cloth and apply overnight. Do several nights in a row.

Ankles and legs

Potato peelings—take a handful of unsprayed potato peelings and cover with 2 cups of water. Simmer 15 minutes and strain. Take 2 tablespoons of this in 1 glass of water. Drink 4 glasses a day for 14 days. After several days, legs and ankles should be normal size.

T

TAPEWORM
Pomegranate

TEARS
Excessive
B_2.

Not enough
B_1.

TENSION
Carrot seeds
Make a tea of carrot seeds and drink a cup now and then. It will take tension from the smooth muscles, such as the intestines.

TOBACCO CRAVING
Laurel leaves
Make a tea and also put in soups or meat dishes.

(*See also* STOP SMOKING)

TOE
Sour cherries
For gout inflammation of big toe, 15 sour cherries in the morning for 3 weeks.

TONGUE
Tongue adheres to roof of mouth
>Nutmeg.

Mapped when red, scraped patches appear
>Dandelion root or leaves.

Deep red
>Niacin, B-complex.

Fissures
>B_2.

Purple red
>B_2.

Yellow or white
>Put mint leaves on tongue.

TONSILS
Banana
>Banana baked in the skin and mashed with a little fresh cream or olive oil for swollen tonsils. Make compresses.

Grapefruit juice

TOOTH, BLEEDING
Black tea
>After extraction take one Lipton black tea bag and wet it in warm water and apply.

TOOTH DECAY
>Boil 1 cup of chopped mulberry bark or fine twigs in 1 quart concord grape juice for $1/2$ hour. Take 1 tablespoon 6 times daily. Keep it in your mouth, then swallow.

TOOTH, LOOSE
Apple cider vinegar
>Hold warm apple cider vinegar in your mouth, spit it out. Do this several times a day. Or boil sage with honey.

Parsley
>3 cups parsley tea daily.

TOOTH POWDER
Soda and salt

TOOTHACHE
Black tea
> Soak a black tea bag in hot water, apply to cheek.

Hyssop
> Between tooth and gum overnight

Cloves
> A little oil of clove inserted in the cavity. Powdered milk in the hole will stop the toothache for a while also.

Pepper and mustard
> Place on a piece of cloth and put over aching cheek.

TRANQUILIZER
Sesame seeds
> For sound nerves take ½ cup sesame seeds, blend in 2 cups water, and add 3 tablespoons whey. A little honey makes it delicious.

TUMOR (fatty)
Asparagus
> Buy a can of asparagus—the cheap ones are the best. Blend it and take 2 tablespoons in the morning and 2 tablespoons at night. Put it on bread or eat alone.

Bible remedy
> Take 1 pound white figs in 3 quarts milk, boil until well done. Place figs in a blender, make a poultice out of it, and apply to tumor overnight. Renew this every 12 hours for 3 days. Also drink ½ cup of this fig milk 3 times daily.

U

ULCER DIET
If you are in a hurry to be healed from stomach ulcers, follow the carrot diet:
> Boil a good portion of carrots in pure water without aluminum of any kind (pots, pans, or foil). When the carrots are done you eat them in different styles:

Take a napkin and eat them rabbit style.
Mash them to puree.
Broil them after they are cooked.
Make a soup pureed.
Slice them lengthwise or square.

No butter, no salt. That is all you eat for 7 days. Twice a day you may have 6 ounces raw carrot juice, either with 2 tablespoons cream or with 6 ounces goat's milk.

ULCERATED COLITIS
Homeopathic *Thuja occidentalis*, goldenseal

ULCERATED INTESTINES
Potatoes, garlic, goldenseal

ULCERATED SKIN
White pond lily

Wounds
>Warm milk compresses—the bacteria are drawn into the milk compresses and the infected wounds can heal.

ULCERATED STOMACH
Okra, apples, string beans

UREMIA
Epsom salts drink
>1 teaspoon Epsom salts in 7 ounces water every hour for 4 hours.

URIC ACID
Sour cherries
>Balancer.

Hydrangea
>Deposit.

Melon
>Watermelon or muskmelon will straighten out uric acid.

Asparagus, cranberries, spinach, endive, and watercress
>3 servings a day, must be cooked on low heat.

URINATION
Pain: white urination

>1 teaspoon marjoram in 8 ounces water, simmer 10 minutes, sweeten with brown sugar. Place a handful of parsley over the bladder.

Blood in urine

>1 quart water, 4 ounces juniper berries, boil for 10 minutes, take $\frac{1}{2}$ cup 4 times daily.

UTERUS (hemorrhage)
Ice

>Ice to nipples will stop uterus bleeding at once.

V

VASCULAR CONGESTION
Whey

>When one makes yogurt or cheese there is a transparent liquid released. This is whey. Whey removes vascular congestion and is a mind booster.

VASODILATATION
Garlic

VEINS, ENLARGED
Horse chestnut

VEINS, VARICOSE
Cottage cheese

>Take cottage cheese and spread it on a cloth as you would spread butter on bread. Cover with another cloth and apply over aching and unsightly veins all night if possible, or just several hours. Do this every night until gone.

Cabbage
>Grate and fill up a piece of cheesecloth. Tie over your painful areas and let sit overnight. You also may take lettuce leaves (head lettuce works the best) and do the same.

Sage

VERTIGO
Violet leaves

Daisy tea
>In elderly.

Crab apples
>Boil crab apples and eat 1 teaspoon every day.

VIRAL INFECTION
Lettuce, basil

Lettuce water
>Take leaf lettuce and boil in water, drink 4 ounces every hour.

VISION, DIMNESS
Linden flower, carrot juice, *Kidney Tea*

VISION, OBJECTS LOOK DISTORTED IN SIZE
Nutmeg
>$1/4$ teaspoon in 6 ounces of hot water.

VITAMIN A
>Cannot work without iodine.
>The liver needs iodine. The liver also makes molecules of energy out of vitamin A.
>Carrot juice is vitamin A plus iodine.
>Hyperglycemia—no carrot juice.
>Allergic to eggs: vitamin A.
>Some people think they are allergic to eggs when a substance in eggs creates too much insulin.

VITAMIN C REPLACEMENT
Alfalfa seed

Cranberry juice
>Frequently recommended for people whose body is not utilizing vitamin C properly. The best time to drink it is early afternoon. Make sure you drink cranberry juice and not Cranapple or the other mixes.

VOMITING OF FOOD (chronic)

Vinegar

> In case of severe vomiting moisten a cloth with warm vinegar and apply over abdomen.

Dill seed

> $^1/_2$ teaspoon dill seed in water or chew it.

WATER RETENTION

Fennel, watermelon seed tea, parsley tea

WEAK

Digestion

> *Anacardium occidentale* (cashew nut).

Joints

> Ginger tea.

Ligaments

> Potassium, E, C.

Memory

> Club moss.

Muscles

> *Alchemilla vulgaris* (lady's mantle).

Stomach

> Rosemary, sorrel.

Willed

> Sesame seeds.

Woman (weakness in)

> Potassium.

Sesame seeds

> They are a complete amino acid supplier and make strong willed people. They supply osmium, a trace mineral.

WHOOPING COUGH

B$_6$, red clover

Also, rub onion juice into soles of feet or into the back. Or ginger tea or 1 tablespoon thyme, boil in 1 cup water for 20 minutes, strain, add honey, take 1 teaspoon every hour.

WICKEDNESS

Anacardium occidentale (cashew nut)

WOMEN WITH BITING DISPOSITIONS

Cramp bark

WORMS

In general

White figs are useful for de-worming. Figs and fig juice paralyze any worm, even the tapeworm, pinworm, and roundworm.

Garlic

Cut 3 cloves of garlic. Boil in 8 ounces of milk for 5 minutes, let cool so you can drink it. Do this before going to sleep for 10 days in a row.

Pomegranate

As juice or eaten raw, it is a great help to keep worms out of the system.

Pumpkin seeds

Eat $1/2$ cup pumpkin seeds a day, especially before a meal on an empty stomach. Worms are stripped from their protective skins by pumpkin seeds.

Figs

Eat 3 or 4 figs 2 times daily.

SPECIFIC HEALING PROPERTIES IN FOODS

ANISE   For flatulent conditions.

APPLES   Whatever ails you: gall bladder trouble, liver
                         trouble, diarrhea, tooth decay, constipation, loss
                         of appetite; good as poultices, too. When some-
                         one is very ill, take an apple and scrape the
                         meat with a silver spoon. You will see them
                         return.

APRICOTS   Detoxifies the liver and pancreas.

ASPARAGUS   For fatty tumors and the like. Helpful in urinary
                         secretions.

AVOCADO   A fat and protein supplier. Good for the diabetic.

BARLEY   A calcium supplier, colon aid, and lymph
                         cleanser.

BEANS (adzuki)   For kidney trouble and swollen ankles.

BEANS (green)   Remove metallic poison. Good for the malfunc-
                         tions of the pancreas.

BEANS (lima)   Make a dish with lima beans, bell peppers, and
                         sweet potato to combat drug residue.

BEANS (red)   Build muscles. Served with corn, a complete
                         protein.

BEANS (white)   For the eyes and for liver trouble.

BEANS and CORN   Muscle builders.

BEEF	Muscle food.
BEETS	Spleen food.
BELL PEPPER	Eyes and digestion (increases pepsin).
BLACK BEAN JUICE	For hoarseness and laryngitis.
BLACKBERRIES	Colon food. For diarrhea.
BLACKSTRAP MOLASSES	A mineral and iron supplier.
BLUEBERRIES	Pancreas food. For sugar problems.
BLUEBERRY and BANANA	Pancreatitis.
BUCKWHEAT	For energy and warmth. For strong muscles.
BUTTERNUT	Liver food.
CABBAGE	For vitamin U, the tissue builder.
CARROTS	Eyes, blood, and lymph.
CELERY	A low calorie reducing aid.
CELERY SEED	Drink the tea for obesity.
CHERRIES	For gout.
CHERRIES (sour)	For gout and as a blood cleanser.
CHICKEN	A gland food.
CHICKPEAS	A gland food. Good protein. An anti-virus, particularly anti-polio virus.
CRAB APPLE	For vertigo.

CRANBERRY	A kidney food. Releases sudden cramps as in asthma and the like.
CUCUMBER	A skin remedy, kidney cleanser, and infection cleanser.
CURRANTS	Builds resistance to colds. For anemia.
EGGPLANT	Give the peelings and dulse to the afflicted tumor.
FIGS	A de-wormer.
FISH	Good protein and iodine supplier.
GARLIC	Carbohydrate residue in tissue and glands.
GRAPEFRUIT	A lime supplier. A flu destroyer.
GRAPES	Antitumor, good for anemia, and an aura builder.
INDIAN CORN	Perfect food for man. Has all the energies, amino acids, and hormones the body needs.
KALE	For resistance to colds.
LEEK	For reducing. A pancreas food, tissue builder, and brain food.
LEMON	Vitamin C.
LEMON (white of rind)	Bioflavonoid. Strengthens tissue.
LENTILS	Iron. Contains protein supplies of the best quality.
LIME	For yellow jaundice.
MEAT	Lots of calories. Protein that gives an explosive energy. Appetite satisfying.

MILLET	Meat of the vegetarian. Fifteen percent protein.
OATS	Brain food.
OILS, COLD PRESSED	Needed to assimilate the proteins from vegetables. Also a kidney food.
OKRA	Regulates female bleeding. Gives strength to leukemic patients.
OKRA and APPLES	For ulceration of the stomach.
ONION	Make a soup of fresh red and white onions and collards for the flu.
ORANGES	Has vitamin C for flu prevention.
PAPAYA	For protein digestion.
PARSLEY	For piles.
PARSLEY ROOT	For kidneys. When boiled in white wine it is for the heart.
PARSNIP	For intolerance to milk.
PEACHES	Good during pregnancy.
PEARS	Kidney and colon.
PEAS	Green and dried peas are good sources of protein and good for weak stomachs.
PINEAPPLE	Enzyme supplier.
POMEGRANATE	A de-wormer.
POTATO PEELINGS	For kidney ailments.

POTATOES (red)	For stomach and duodenal ulcer.
PRUNES	Iron, constipation.
PUMPKIN	De-wormer, parasites. Spleen and pancreas food.
RADISHES	In small amounts, promote bile flow.
RAISIN	Anemia, blood builder.
RHUBARB	Colon cleanser.
RICE	Universal acceptance by all tissues (overrated at the present time).
RICE GRUEL	Diarrhea.
ROMAINE LETTUCE	Virus infection.
RUTABAGA	Food for prayer. Feeds friendly bacteria in colon. Once a week it would be good.
RYE	Muscle builder.
SAUERKRAUT	Keeps old folks' ailments away.
SESAME SEEDS	Complete amino acid supplier. Makes strong willed people. Supplies osmium, a trace mineral.
SPINACH	Good for you if you have anemia.
STRAWBERRIES	A skin berry.
STRAWBERRIES and SQUASH	Remove metallic poisons, arsenic.
SUNFLOWER SEEDS	Feeds eyes, sinuses, and glands.
SWEET POTATO	Gland food.

SWISS CHARD	Arthritis (contains Wulzen factor).
TOMATO	As poultices in deep rooted afflictions. When stewed, good for liver. Fresh tomatoes are a vitamin C supplier. Green tomatoes in very small quantities are a gland stimulant. Always remove the core of the stem. Make a deep insertion. This stem part is poisonous.
TURNIPS	For deep rooted tumors. For deep rooted resentments.
WATERCRESS	Vitamin C and E supplier.
WATERMELON	For sluggish kidney and a kidney cleanser.

Books by Hanna

"Wholistic health represents an attitude toward well being which recognizes that we are not just a collection of mechanical parts, but an integrated system which is physical, mental, social and spiritual."

Ageless Remedies from Mother's Kitchen

You will laugh and be amazed at all that you can do in your own pharmacy, the kitchen. These time tested treasures are in an easy to read, cross referenced guide. (94 pages)

Allergy Baking Recipes

Easy and tasty recipes for cookies, cakes, muffins, pancakes, breads and pie crusts. Includes wheat free recipes, egg and milk free recipes (and combinations thereof) and egg and milk substitutes. (34 pages)

Alzheimer's Science and God

This little booklet provides a closer look at this disease and presents Hanna's unique, religious perspectives on Alzheimer's disease. (15 pages)

Arteriosclerosis and Herbal Chelation

A booklet containing information on Arteriosclerosis causes, symptoms and herbal remedies. An introduction to the product *Circu Flow.* (17 pages)

Cancer: Traditional and New Concepts

A fascinating and extremely valuable collection of theories, tests, herbal formulas and special information pertaining to many facets of this dreaded disease. (65 pages)

Cookbook for Electro-Chemical Energies

The opening of this book describes basic principles of healthy eating along with some fascinating facts you may not have heard before. The rest of this book is loaded with delicious, healthy recipes. A great value. (106 pages)

God Helps Those That Help Themselves

This work is a beautifully comprehensive description of the seven basic physical causes of disease. It is wholistic information as we need it now. A truly valuable volume. (270 pages)

Good Health Through Special Diets

This book shows detailed outlines of different diets for different needs. Dr. Reidlin, M.D. said, "The road to health goes through the kitchen not through the drug store," and that's what this book is all about. (121 pages)

Hanna's Workshop

A workbook that brings together all of the tools for applying Hanna's testing methods. Designed with 60 templates that enable immediate results.

How to Counteract Environmental Poisons

A wonderful collection of notes and information gleaned from many years of Hanna's teachings. This concise and valuable book discusses many toxic materials in our environment and shows you how to protect yourself from them. It also presents Hanna's insights on how to protect yourself, your family and your community from spiritual dangers. (53 pages)

Instant Herbal Locator

This is the herbal book for the do-it-yourself person. This book is an easy cross referenced guide listing complaints and the herbs that do the job. Very helpful to have on hand. (122 pages)

Instant Vitamin-Mineral Locator

A handy, comprehensive guide to the nutritive values of vitamins and minerals. Used to determine bodily deficiencies of these essential elements and combinations thereof, and what to do about these deficiencies. According to your symptoms, locate your vitamin and mineral needs. A very helpful guide. (55 pages)

New Dimensions in Healing Yourself

The consummate collection of Hanna's teachings. An unequated volume that compliments all of her other books as well as her years of teaching. (155 pages)

Old Time Remedies for Modern Ailments

A collection of natural remedies from Eastern and Western cultures. There are 20 fast cleansing methods and many ways to rebuild your health. A health classic. (115 pages)

Parasites: The Enemy Within

A compilation of years of Hanna's studies with parasites. A rare treasure and one of the efforts to expose the truths that face us every day. (62 pages)

The Pendulum, the Bible and Your Survival

A guide booklet for learning to use a pendulum. Explains various aspects of energies, vibrations and forces. (22 pages)

The Seven Spiritual Causes of Ill Health

This book beautifully reveals how our spiritual and emotional states have a profound effect on our physical well being. It addresses fascinating topics such as karma, gratitude, trauma, laughter as medicine . . . and so much more. A wonderful volume full of timeless treasures. (145 pages)

Spices to the Rescue

This is a great resource for how our culinary spices can enrich our health and offer first aid from our kitchen. Filled with insightful historical references. (64 pages)

Attention

Soma Board

To protect our families from environmental poisons we need two devices in our kitchen.

The first one is the *Soma Board.* It is a unique invention in the field of Ether-Technology. It is a flat board. On this you place your food, milk, juice, or water for just a minute or two.

The device will neutralize the residues of:

> chemicals
> pesticides
> preservatives
> metals

that might be attached to your groceries. The wholesomeness of your food improves and it tastes a lot better.

I have used this board for years and my family stays clear of environmental poisons.

Pico Board Angel Help

The second device is the *Pico Board* or Angel Help. It is a flat box on which you place your food and drink. The device will counteract the vibrations of cesium 137, cobalt 60, and strontium 90 and all the residues caused by irradiating our food. Some of our food is exposed to high levels of gamma radiation. It is a by-product of the nuclear industry. It is said that irradiation of food is harmless. Why then will mice being fed irradiated food not reproduce after the third generation? Why does it make lesions in the brain and all over? I call my device Angel Help. Working as an entire congregation, the members of the Chapel of Miracles came up with this device.

Both devices are priced very reasonably.